How to Help Your Child Overcome Bedwetting

Alicia White

TABLE OF CONTENTS

1

INTRODUCTION

When bed-wetting becomes a problem in your home, what do you do?

Often times when a child is wetting his or her bed, the reason is due either to an undiagnosed medical condition or due to psychological effects. As a parent, you will want to find out what is happening with your child so that you can stop bedwetting.

Unfortunately, there are things that prevent many parents from trying to determine what causes their child's bedwetting. Some of the things that stop parents from helping their children include:

- Shame (parents worry that a child's bedwetting will reflect badly on them while children may be reluctant to speak with a pediatrician about a problem that is embarrassing for them).

- Misconceptions about bedwetting

- Time (some parents may be reluctant to take the time to help a child, assuming that bedwetting is a normal childhood ailment and will be resolved by itself)

- Anger (parents may feel frustrated or angry with the problem and this may make them think of the problem as unimportant)

Thanks to the fact that the book is organized into tips, you can easily read the book a tip or two at a time, in your spare time, and try several ideas that may be effective in stopping bedwetting. Plus, in this book you will be given the facts about bedwetting, and the latest research and information you need to make educated choices that can help your child stop wetting the bed.

Before we start to consider some of the things that can be done to stop bedwetting in its tracks, we need to discuss the very idea of bedwetting. Bedwetting occurs at night, and often in children who have no trouble or little trouble controlling their bladder during the day. This means that for these children, bedwetting makes bedtime a terrible time.

Rather than being a time of stories and rest, bedtime becomes a time of conflict and stress for both parent and child.

Bedwetting is not a rare problem. Experts think that five to seven million children in this country wet the bed at least occasionally. The older children get, the less likely they are to wet the bed, as children outgrow the problem at a rate of roughly 15% per year.

However, this means that 1% of older teenagers, and 20% of children between the ages of six and five will still wet their bed regularly.

Bedwetting creates stress for the entire family. Parents may be frustrated and fatigued by the washing of sheets, drying of mattresses, and reassurances that follow each incident of bedwetting.

The medical term for bedwetting is Enuresis and it is a serious subject for medical research. Researchers have found that a few basic causes of bedwetting seem to be the culprit for most sufferers of Enuresis. Among medical causes, ailments such as urinary tract infections, allergies, diabetes, cell anemia and sleep disorders are often the culprit.

Since bedwetting is often the first sign of these problems, it is a good idea to get your child checked out for these conditions. In addition, researchers have found that psychological reasons such as stress, upset, and trauma often contribute to bedwetting.

Children who wet the bed for any reason often suffer needlessly, and this suffering is the best reason to get your child help for Enuresis. Children who wet the bed often suffer from low self-esteem, withdrawal, stress, fear, and other problems. These children may suffer from sleeplessness because they fear or are embarrassed by what happens when they sleep.

A child with Enuresis is often teased by others and may feel dirty by the smell of urine about them. The child may even avoid others out of fear of ridicule. At the very least, fun childhood activities such as camp, sleep overs, and camping may be made into traumatic rather than happy events for the bedwetting child.

Many parents wonder whether they should seek help for bedwetting. After all, despite the problems of bedwetting, many doctors still recommend patience and time as the best way to resolve bedwetting, as many children overcome the problem with no extra help.

Of course, many children does not mean all children, and telling an anxious child that he or she will wake up dry "someday" is not terribly reassuring for anyone. In general, there are a few signs that you should seek help for bedwetting:

- You child asks for help. If your child thinks that bedwetting is enough of a problem that they need help with it, then bedwetting is serious enough to demand some sort of remedy. Period.

- Your child has suddenly developed a problem after having no problems staying dry before. Often, this is a sign of some problem and should be investigated.

- Your child acts out or has problems with others (teasing or lack of friends) as a result of bedwetting.

- Your child avoids normal activities that they like (camping, going out) because of bedwetting.

- Child is bedwetting regularly after eight years old and the problem is causing distress.

- Bedwetting is causing problems in the household.

If any of the following apply, then consider the following 101 tips - you are sure to find solutions to try for you and your child!

2

INITIAL TIPS FOR DEALING WITH BEDWETTING IN YOUR HOUSEHOLD

There are some tips you will want to adopt right away in order to deal with bedwetting in your household:

Tip #1: Work on Sensitivity

One of the biggest impacts of bedwetting on your child is an emotional one, so you should work on making sure that your household is sensitive to your child's situation. No one at home should tease your child or make them feel terrible about their bedwetting. The more teased a child is about bedwetting, the more difficult it will be for the child to overcome the problem.

The older a child is, the more ashamed they may be of wetting the bed, and the more important it will be to stay level-headed and calm to prevent shaming the child. Shaming will only result in trauma and may even make bedwetting worse.

Tip #2: Watch your own sensitivity levels.

It is not just siblings and other children that need to be considered. Parents often inadvertently are insensitive to their child's bedwetting. They are frustrated by the laundry that must be done and are sometimes even angered by having so many sheets stained or even ruined by urine.

On a rushed morning, dealing with urine-soaked sheets before dashing off to work can be frustrating, but it is crucial not to lose your temper. Even if you manage to be calm most of the time, one outburst about bedwetting will linger in your child's mind and make them feel ashamed.

If you find that you have no time to deal with sheets and clean-up in the morning, strip the sheets and leave them for later. If you are angry by the cost of bed linens, consider buying less expensive sheets in bulk for a while to reduce costs for yourself. Keep rags and other clean up items (deodorizer and cleaner) in the child's room for fast cleaning.

Work on reducing your stress levels when it comes to bedwetting, and you are less likely to make an unfortunate comment from pure stress.

Tip #3: Educate Yourself

Throughout this ebook, you will be able to educate yourself about the facts of bedwetting. However, you will want to share what you have learned with others in your household. If you have several children, you need to be aware that siblings will often tease a brother or sister who "still wets the bed." Letting these children know that Enuresis is a condition can help them be more sensitive towards their sibling while measures are taken to prevent bedwetting.

Tip #4: Educate your child

For the child affected by Enuresis, being told the facts about bedwetting can be a big help. Children often hear misconceptions about bedwetting from other children. Myths such as "only babies wet the bed" can be hurtful to your child and can make him or her feel as though there is something "wrong" with them.

Often, explaining that Enuresis is an actual condition and talking about the remedies doctors have come up for it can help persuade your child that bedwetting is curable and a common problem. That way, your child can focus on resolving the problem rather than worry about the embarrassment they feel.

Tip #5: Visit a Doctor

Since some bedwetting is caused by undiagnosed medical conditions such as diabetes or allergies, it makes sense to take your child to a doctor to be checked out. If there is a doctor in your area who is known for treating children with Enuresis, so much the better. In either case, ruling out medical problems can be a big relief. If a medical problem is causing your child to wet the bed, coping with the problem will also generally resolve the Enuresis.

Tip #6: Evaluate

Evaluate how much of a problem bedwetting is in your family and how often it happens. Frequent bedwetting that causes many tears and embarrassment or even arguments in your household may need more aggressive treatment than bedwetting that occurs once in a while and results in only some extra laundry.

Tip #7: Different types of bedwetting demand different approaches

Also, be sure to differentiate between primary and secondary Enuresis. Primary nocturnal Enuresis is almost never caused by an underlying medical problem. Secondary nocturnal Enuresis means that a child has had control of his or her bladder but has begun wetting the bed.

In these cases, it is especially important to have the child seen by a good pediatrician, as almost all cases of secondary Enuresis are caused by an underlying problem (psychological or physical) and so responds very well to treatment.

Tip #8: Make it less stressful

Once you have evaluated the bedwetting in your household, you can develop a plan of action. Since you will be learning many tips that you can apply to your plan in the upcoming pages, your plan here is basically a contingency plan. On a paper, write down what your child should do when he or she wets the bed.

Ideally, your child should contact you, and then you should take steps to clean up. Share the plan with your child so that when an accident happens, your child can put the plan into action rather than being ashamed and trying to get your attention.

There are also a few things you can do to make bedwetting less stressful. Putting special sheets on your child's bed, for example, can make clean-up much easier. Keeping extra sheets and blankets by your child's room can also make clean-up much faster, especially in a busy household. Even small things you can do to make bedwetting less stressful will allow you and your child to focus on resolving the problem rather than worry about clean up.

This ebook is dedicated to finding and then providing solutions about how to best help and treat the child that wets the bed. As you continue with this ebook, you will find many additional tips for small things that can be done to help make bedwetting less stressful in your home.

Tip #9: Reality Check

Consider whether there really is a problem. Although we often expect kids to grow up fast today, the fact is that occasional bedwetting up to age three is still considered "normal" by most experts - children at this age are still simply learning to do basic things like use the washroom and control their bladder. Even kids up to age five may have an occasional bed wetting "accident" and this should not be a cause for concern. Many experts consider children over five who wet the bed regularly to have nocturnal Enuresis. In many cases, this condition tends to run in families and can last well into teenage years.

Before you start worrying unduly about bedwetting, consider the age of your child. If your child is very young, it may simply take a few months or a year to resolve the issue.

Many children have nighttime accidents until they are five or even older. If your child is older (six, seven, or older), consider whether anyone else in the family suffered from similar bedwetting problems in childhood. Was there something that helped?

Sometimes, just seeing Enuresis as a childhood ailment or a condition in the family that is always resolved eventually can help soothe the frazzled parent and the embarrassed child.

You need to consider the frequency of problems as well. A child who wets the bed after watching a scary movie or before a big day may be less worrisome than the older child who does not seem to be able to sleep through a dry night.

Tip #10: **Once you have calmed down, take action.**

Many of the above tips are intended to get parents and children more comfortable with the bedwetting and accidents that occur when a child is trying to cope with Enuresis.

This is because bedwetting is such a stressful and emotional issue - in fact, some polls have suggested that besides divorce and family conflict, it is one of the most stressful issues for families. Learning to deal with the problem calmly, then, is a big priority.

However, parents should not just allow themselves to be placated into taking no action at all. The fact is, bedwetting can still be a nuisance and a problem for your child, and there are many solutions out there. Once your family has learned to deal with the problem in a level-headed way, do encourage your family to seek solutions rather than wait for the problem to go away on its own. There are many solutions out there that can help your child, so that your son or daughter do not suffer needlessly.

Tip #11: Don't let it become a big deal.

Of course, you want to help your child stop wetting the bed so that they can enjoy a comfortable sleep with no embarrassment in the morning, but be careful that you desire to help does not come across as a sign that there is something wrong. Don't make bedwetting - an un-dangerous condition - become a big issue at your house.

Tip #12: Keep things low-key

Make sure that the approach to bedwetting is a low-key one. Point out that it is not a child's fault and that it usually means that a child simply needs to keep growing up - there is nothing abnormal about it. It often helps if the child knows that others in the family have experienced bedwetting and have grown out of it.

Also, make sure that any treatments or remedies used are offered in a low-key, non- threatening way. There is no need to keep stressing the child's bedwetting throughout the day. Offer some therapy during the day but allow the child to play and just enjoy being a kid.

Tip #13: Let the child tell you when he or she has wet the bed.

If your child wets the bed, make sure that siblings or other well-intentioned members of the household don't announce "Johnny wet the bed -again." This just leads to shaming.

Instead, it is often helpful to have a quiet time in the morning when your child can tell you himself or herself. Having a system (such as a calendar where the child marks wet and dry nights) can make it easier for the child to approach you, as there is a routine for sharing this information.

Tip #14: Let the child help.

If it will help your child feel less embarrassed, let him or her help clean up. He or she can tidy up the pillows or fold the sheets. In some cases, this can make the child feel less inept and babyish, if they can be entrusted with a grownup chore. Plus, if they can help clean the bed they may feel in control of a small part of their bedwetting.

Do not make cleaning up a punishment, but rather offer it as a way to make the child more comfortable. A comment such as "would you like to put the pillowcases on the pillows to make your bed more comfortable?" makes it clear that the child is not being punished for wetting the bed.

Tip #15:   Stay alert for bigger problems

In the big scheme of things, bedwetting is not a big problem. Your child is not in any danger of serious injury or harm if he or she occasionally or even regularly loses control of their bladder at night. To a child, however, it may not seem like a small problem. For this reason, as a parent, you must remain alert for signs of bigger problems.

If your child's bedwetting causes them to feel so ashamed or upset that their regular lie is affected, then that is a serious problem. If their schoolwork is affected, then their bedwetting may affect their development as well. If children are bullying or teasing your child to the point that social activities are a problem, then your child may experience alarming signs of stress and depression. In any of these cases, swift action is needed to ensure that your child stays safe and happy.

If your child shows any of the following symptoms, he or she may be struggling more than you know and should be taken to a doctor or pediatrician to get help sorting out the emotions he or she could be felling:

- Sudden and big changes in appetite (eats a lot less or far more)
- Fearful or withdrawn with others
- Does not show interest in regular activities

- Does not spend time with others and does not want to spend time with others

- Cries, gets angry or is very quiet often

- Mood swings

- Trouble sleeping

- Loss of control of bladder during the day

- Grades dramatically worsen

- Bruising on the body or favorite toys are broken (may indicate bullying or self- destructive behavior)

If you notice these problems, you will want to seek more aggressive treatment for the bedwetting and you will want to visit a doctor or counselor to help your child deal with the problems caused by bedwetting.

Tip #16:	**Make sure that no medication is causing the problem.**

Check the side effects and directions on your child's medication. If your child is taking any medications that cause extreme drowsiness or an urgent need to urinate, the medications may be causing the problem. Medications that make your child very tired may simply not allow your child's body to wake him or her up in time to go to the bathroom.

Talk to your pharmacist or doctor about any medication your child is taking and ask whether the substances may add to the bedwetting problem. Of course, your child may need medication that does not help his or her bedwetting, but in some cases doses or medications can be changed in order to prevent such side effects.

Tip #17: **Make sure that your child has easy access to a bathroom.**

A bright night light and a bathroom that is easy to access quickly at night will go a long way towards making sure that your child can get to the bathroom in time. Not every household can arrange to provide a bathroom near a child's bedroom, but consider sleeping arrangements closely and consider rearrangements that could make nighttime bathroom trips much easier. Even something as simple as moving your child's bed closer to the bedroom door can save a few seconds at night, reducing accidents.

Tip #18: **Get your child to go to sleep a bit earlier.**

Children who are tired may have a hard time waking up for anything - including a full bladder. If your child gets the sleep he or she needs, they will not be so overtired that they will be unable to wake up.

Tip #19: **Look for psychological triggers.**

Emotional states often add to bedwetting or even trigger it. If your child is undergoing an upset (divorce in the family, death in the family, bullying, moving, conflicts with siblings) this may contribute to bedwetting. In these cases, you can either wait for the child to adjust (at which point the bedwetting may cease too) or you can have your child see a pediatrician or child therapist. Sometimes, even talking about the problems can help, so be sure to discuss anything that seems to be bothering your child.

Tip #20: Have Your child self-monitor

Once you develop a system for dealing with bedwetting, or once you and your family start trying to control bedwetting in some way, it is useful to have a child check off on a calendar which nights were completely dry, on which nights a bathroom was reached successfully, and which nights were wet. Keeping track lets your child get involved in the solution process, which will make your child feel more confident. Once your child sees any improvement, he or she will likely be encouraged to further success.

Tip #21: Care for your child's skin.

Bedwetting has few serious side effects, but one of the physical discomforts it may cause is skin problems. Urine is a mix of fluid and waste chemicals from the body. When left on skin for a few hours in the night, it can irritate. Skin may appear red initially, and may turn sore and flaky if the skin is not treated. The skin will also thicken if the irritation is not treated, eventually turning wrinkled and pale. Although not dangerous, this type of skin irritation can be very painful for a child.

Skin problems can affect any child who wets the bed, but the problem is more aggravated in those who wet the bed often and in those who wear absorbent products to collect the urine. Genitals and buttocks can be affected. In those who wear absorbent underpants, the leg bands and waist bands are often the most irritated.

Once bedwetting is resolved, the rash and skin irritation it causes will disappear as well. Until your child has stopped wetting the bed, though, you can try to reduce the skin irritation the problem causes. To prevent skin rashes and soreness:

- Make sure the child washes each morning, especially after a "wet" night. The skin affected by the area should be especially well washed using a mild and moisturizing soap.

- Encourage your child to rinse the buttocks and genital area when changing absorbent underpants and after waking up after having wet the bed.

- Use a very soft sponge - not a harsh washcloth - on any irritated skin area

- Some parents find that applying petroleum ointment to affected areas and areas affected by urine is helpful

- Choose correct-fitting absorbent undergarments, if your child uses them. Make sure that the waist band and the leg bands are not too snug. Choose the most absorbent type you can and look for a brand that offers a top layer that keeps moisture away from the skin.

- Talk to your pediatrician if skin irritation continues. He or she may be able to offer a medicated cream to soothe sore skin.

Tip #22: Get your child's consent.

As you continue to read through this ebook, you will find many tips for dealing with bedwetting. Some of these will seem like great ideas to you and you will likely want to put them into effect right away. However, you should be careful about choosing bedwetting solutions, for any remedy you choose needs to have your child's consent.

Many well-intentioned parents rush out to buy the latest gadget or device for treating bedwetting or for making it less of a problem only to be horrified to learn that their children want nothing to do with the expensive method.

It is important not to force a method on a child. It is completely ineffective as in some cases (such as behavior modification) you actually need your child's enthusiasm and participation for a method to work. In other cases, forcing a bedwetting remedy on a child will be ineffective and can actually lead to more bedwetting because of all the stress caused by the "supposed remedy."

Also, in saying that they don't "like" a remedy children may be trying to say something more - such as that the remedy is uncomfortable or causes more embarrassment that the bedwetting itself.

Tip #23: Work with your child in resolving bedwetting.

When you approach a child with a way or resolving bedwetting, you can often ensure a better reception by approaching the subject in a sensitive and informative way. Explain to your child what the method involves, answer any questions, and express that it may help him or her with bedwetting. Make sure that you explain whether a method is temporary, as a child will be more likely to accept something new for a little while, or on a trial basis, rather than accept something for a longer time.

3

BEHAVIOR MODIFICATION

Behavior modification simply means that you train your child or teach your child to wake up in time to go to the bathroom. Behavior modification is considered the most effective way to help a child with bedwetting, as it actually teaches a child to wake up "in time" rather than just treating the symptoms of bedwetting.

Parents should not take "behavior modification" to mean that bedwetting is a behavioral problem that needs rigorous correction to fix. Nothing could be further from the truth. Rather, behavior modification works more by teaching your child the nighttime bladder control that most children learn sooner or later. There are many types of behavior modification tips that have been proven effective in helping children overcome bedwetting:

Tip #24: Discipline Will Not Work

Many years ago, it was thought that children who wet the bed were simply poorly taught, were developmentally delayed (or otherwise "abnormal") or just needed more discipline.

Even though most parents know better today, many still look at bedwetting as a way of "acting out."

It is important not to discipline your child for wetting the bed. This method not only does not work, but the stress of the discipline may make the problem worse. No child wants to wet the bed after everyone else can stay "dry" for the night. The child who has a hard time not wetting the bed needs sympathy and help, not discipline.

Tip #25: Offer Positive Reinforcement and Praise

When your child makes it through nights without wetting the bed, be sure to offer praise. Not only will this help the child if he or she feels bad when accidents happen, but it will subconsciously motivate your child to continue trying to correct the problem as well. A system as simple as offering gold stars is effective. A week that is dry should be given a slightly larger treat.

You can also use a points system. Have each star or dry night count for a point. When your child reaches three points, allow him or her to have a small treat. Five points can mean a very small gift. Ten points can mean a trip someplace fun, and so on. Keep points posted where they are visible. The excitement generated by this system will

21

encourage your child to keep trying and press on.

Tip #26: Give your child hope that the problem is not forever

If your child seems to be doing better, remind him or her again that most people overcome bedwetting with time and notice that their situation seems to improving itself.

A child who does not believe that the problem will improve will simply have a harder time with the problem and for such a child the problem will seem larger and more dire than it really is. Help your child see that bedwetting will be resolved and your child will be calmer, happier, and so more able to work with you to get help for Enuresis.

Tip #27: Focus on Normal Bladder Control

Most children who wet the bed have trouble at night. However, a small percentage of children have overactive bladders, which means that they frequently have to go to the bathroom and may even have a hard time controlling their bladder during the daytime. If this describes your child, take him or her to a doctor or urologist to see what treatments are available for your child's overactive bladder.

If your child only has trouble with control over the night, then it may be a good idea to focus on the fact that your child does do well in going to the bathroom during the day.

Offer your child encouragement by pointing out that he or she can make it to the bathroom during the day and reassure your child that most people learn to control as well in the night, as well.

Tip #28:   Night lifting

Night lifting is a technique that requires the parent to wake up the child in the night. Most children lose control of their bladder at a similar time each night (this is especially true if the child follows the same routine each day). If you can note when each accident occurs, you can set your alarm before this time, wake your child up, and lead them to the bathroom.

You can also try waking yourself and your child up twice a night. In many cases, this helps the child wake dry and encourages the child to keep trying to wake up before they are woken up. However, children may resist waking up in the night, especially if they are tired.

Tip #29:   Bladder Control Exercises

Your doctor may prescribe exercises for your child to help him or her control their bladder more effectively. Some patients with Enuresis benefit from holding their urine as long as possible before releasing. The idea is to keep repeating these exercises in order to help the body develop more control.

Bladder control exercise:

1) Have your child tell you when he or she has to "go" during the day.

2) Explain to your child that you are doing an exercise to help

him or her stay dry at night. Have the child hold the urine.

3) Have your child go to the washroom

4) Repeat daily, slowly increasing the amount of time you make your child wait

Tip #30: Urination control exercise

Some doctors find that helping the child control urination helps control the urinary sphincter, or the muscle that holds back or releases urine. This exercise is often used in conjunction with the bladder control exercise and is completely safe.

Urine Control exercise:

1) When your child urinates, have your child stop urinating "mid-stream" - that is, have your child start urinating and then stop by squeezing the muscles (urinary sphincter) that control the flow of urine.

2) Have your child start-stop three times.

3) Repeat process during each bathroom visit.

Some parents find the two exercises above useful. The idea is that the child will control the bladder more effectively during the day, causing the control to be present at night, as well.

In general, these exercises work best with children over the age of six years and those who are willing to work hard to control their bladder. Some small improvement should be visible in about two weeks.

Tip #31: Try Visualization

Visualization is a behavior modification tool that has proven effective in helping people accomplish many things, from waking up without an alarm to quitting smoking. You can use the same technique to help your child overcome bedwetting:

1) To begin, have your child relax and close their eyes. You should be in a quiet and comfortable room that has few distractions. Your child should be sitting down or lying down. Have your child breathe deeply and relax.

2) Now, have your child imagine sleeping in their regular bed and in their regular sleep wear.

3) Next, have then imagine having to go to the washroom. Your child should really imagine the pressure of having to urinate. Ask your child to imagine what it feels like to have to "go" during the day and have your child imagine that same feeling as vividly as possible in their imagining of the sleep.

4) Now, have your child imagine waking up and going to the washroom.

Have your child imagine this several times over a period of time. People who use visualization sometimes practice seeing a goal several times a day for weeks. Experts think that visualization works by having the body imagine how things are to be done so precisely and intensely that the body actually accepts the mind's visual clues as reality.

The body actually believes what has been visualized is real. If your child imagines waking up in time to go to the bathroom, then, he or she will have set a sort or emotional and mental precedent for doing so in reality. Visualization is especially effective with older children and can be used with other behavior modification techniques. It is very safe and will generally show results in about two weeks.

Tip #32:   Avoid lots of fluids before bed

It is important to keep your child hydrated. Drinking enough water helps the body function properly and helps keep the kidneys healthy. However, encouraging your child to drink most of his or her water intake earlier in the day so that less water is drunk in the hour or two before bedtime can help ensure that the body does not produce lots of urine at night.

Remember, though: Encourage your child to drink more fluids, not less, even if it does mean some wet nights. Drinking fluids helps the bladder and kidney function well, which will help ensure dry nights in the long run. Dehydration and lack of fluids will not solve anything, and may make the problem worse as people with smaller bladder retention have a harder time staying dry at night.

Tip #33:   Watch what fluids your child drinks

Some fluids cause more problems that others. While your child is trying to overcome bedwetting, it is often best to stick with water. Colas, dark teas, and coffee all contain caffeine that irritates the bladder and also may increase the urgency to urinate more frequently.

If your child is older, alcohol may also affect bedwetting by ensuring that motor controls (needed to wake up) are affected while the need to urinate is increased.

Apple juice also seems to cause increased urine in some children, thanks to the two substances, patulin and gallic acid, that it contains. Encourage your child to eat apples during the day, but do not serve apple juice or applesauce in the evenings.

Tip #34:   Watch what your child consumes

Some parents have also found that sugary foods, carbonated drinks, milk, yellow cheese and other products containing these foods. Try cutting specific foods from your child's diet for a while to see whether these foods have any effect on bedwetting. Monitor what your child eats before bedtime closely and eliminate any foods that seem to contribute to bedwetting, or at least limit these foods to morning.

Remember: When limiting specific foods, take great care to ensure that you child eats a balanced diet that still includes plenty of foods from each food group. Bedwetting is a minor problem compared to vitamin deficiency.

Tip #35:   Night trips to the bathroom.

Encourage your child to go to the bathroom before sleep. You can even wake him or her up when you go to sleep so that he or she can urinate again. This gets rid of the urine in the bladder, reducing the chances that the bladder will be left with enough urine to vacate in the night again. Even if your child wets the bed, the amount of wetness will be reduced. Some parents also find that this technique alone is enough to help bedwetting. Even if it is not, it is a safe method that can be used with other remedies.

Tip #36: Wake up alarm

For many children who wet the bed, the problem comes from the fact that the bladder simply does not communicate well with the body. For most of us, when we have to urinate during sleep, our body wakes us up and we can head to the bathroom before returning to bed. For children with Enuresis, this system does not work. In addition, many children who wet the bed are also very heavy sleepers. Basically, the bladder empties itself since the body does not wake up to allow the child to go to the bathroom. In some cases, the child might not even notice the problem until they wake up the next morning.

There are a number of alarms on the market that your child can wear. These emit a noise when moisture is detected. They will wake your child up, allowing him or her to go to the bathroom. Even if your child is a very heavy sleeper and will not wake up, the alarm can wake up the rest of the household, so that you can wake your child up. The idea behind this device is that the child will eventually learn to wake him or herself after being woken up by the alarm several times. Some improvement will usually be seen in about two weeks.

4

MEDICATION

If your child wets the bed, you will want to try behavior modification first. However, for some children who wet the bed frequently, there are medication options available.

Before deciding to give your child medication, carefully weigh the risks and advantages, as many medications or drugs have side effects:

Tip #37:	DDAVP (Desmopressin Acetate) can help some children

DDAVP is a medication that can help some children stop wetting the bed. This medication works by reducing the amount of urine the body produces at night. DDAVP is based on research which shows that sufferers of Enuresis have lower than normal levels of something called antidiuretic hormone, which is a hormone that regulates the body's urine production by having the kidneys hold water so that less urine flows to the bladder.

Children with low levels of this hormone produce more urine nightly. DDAVP corrects this problem by supplying a substance that works in the body just as the hormone does (to reduce urine) and is also though to help children wake more easily.

It is important to note that Desmopressin Acetate treats the symptoms of bedwetting. This means that while your child is on this medication, they will urinate less during the night. However, the condition of bedwetting per se will not be cured. In many cases, when children stop taking drugs such as DDAVP, bedwetting returns. The hope is that by the time they stop the medication, bedwetting will have passed on its own. This is not always the case.

DDAVP is more likely to work with older children who have normal bladder capacity. Younger children with small bladders are less likely to be helped by the drug.

DDAVP can be taken as a pill or nasal spray. The nasal spray is usually given to younger patients who may have a hard time with the pill form.

However, the spray may be affected by colds or stuffy noses. The pills have also been found to be slightly more effective in some studies.

DDAVP needs to be taken at night but does not need to be taken daily to be effective. This drug also has some side effects, including stomach upset and headache. These symptoms are more common in patients who take the nasal form of the drug. Patients taking the nasal spray may also experience nosebleeds and sinus or nasal pain. More seriously, children who take DDAVP are at risk of seizures caused by water intoxication.

This medical emergency usually has symptoms such as nausea, vomiting and headache. If your child is taking DDAVP and experiences these symptoms, seek medical help right away.

Water intoxication and the risk of seizure can be prevented if children taking DDAVP avoid drinking water the evenings that they are taking the drug. In general, no fluids should be taken in the two hours before retiring and only small amounts in the late afternoon and evening leading up to bedtime.

Tip #38: Imipramine is another drug option.

Imipramine is an anti-depressant which reduces the amount of urine produced during the night. It is sometimes prescribed to children who are unable to take the similarly-working DDAVP, but many doctors are reluctant to prescribe Imipramine because of its many side effects, which can include sleeping problems, nausea, irregular heartbeats, and dry mouth.

Some doctors are also quite cautious with this medication because researchers have not been able to completely define how it works to prevent bedwetting.

Imipramine, like most drugs used to treat bedwetting, works best for older children who have normal bladder capacity. Like most other drugs used to treat the problem, it also only affects symptoms, meaning that those who stop taking Imipramine will frequently resume bedwetting.

This drug is usually taken an hour or two before bedtime. Doses vary based on the patient. Side effects with this medication are rare, but may include irritability, sleeping disruptions, fatigue or drowsiness, changes in appetite, mood swings, and personality changes. It is also possible to die from this drug if an overdose occurs.

Tip #39: **Anticholinergic drugs are an option for some patients.**

Anticholinergic drugs work by increasing bladder capacity and by stopping the contractions of the bladder that some experts think lead to bedwetting. Common Anticholinergic drugs used for bedwetting include oxybutynin (Ditropan) and hyosyamine (Levsinex).

These drugs, unlike many medications used to treat bedwetting, are effective for children with bladder capacity who have trouble controlling their bladders during the daytime as well as at night.

These drugs are usually used with DDAVP for children who wet the bed but may be used alone if a child wets the bed due to general bladder control problems that are present during the day as well. These drugs are taken once or twice a day, often at bedtime. They are not intended for children under twelve years old. Anticholinergic drugs do have a number of side effects, including flushing and dry mouth syndrome.

Tip #40: **Be wary of medicating your child if other options are available.**

The drugs used to treat bedwetting do not cure the problem, and since these drugs also carry risks and side effects, any parent should think carefully and consider all the risks and options before choosing medication. Medication can be useful for children who wet the bed very late or who seem to suffer unduly from the problem. However, medication should never be treated lightly, nor should it be tried as the first method of stopping bedwetting. You should also remember that children who take medication for bedwetting will often revert to bedwetting once the medication has stopped.

5

DEALING WITH YOUR PEDIATRICIAN

Your pediatrician will be an important part of dealing with bedwetting. However, since medical health professionals are so busy today, you will want to make sure that you approach your child's physician in a way that ensures maximum cooperation. Here are some tips that can help you communicate with your child's pediatrician in a way that will ensure better treatment options for your child:

Tip #41: **Keep a diary**

One of the best ways you can help your doctor treat your child is to keep a diary of your child's bedwetting. Starting from the time your child seems to be bedwetting more frequently, keep notes in a small notebook. In this notebook note:

- When your child wets the bed (dates and times, if possible)

- Any family history of bedwetting

- Any results of bedwetting (crying, problems at school, teasing)

- Any medications your child is on or any medical problems your child has had or is having

- Any questions you have about bedwetting

- Any questions or comments your child makes about bedwetting

- Any comments that your child makes before bedtime that may indicate a problem (aches before bed, emotional upsets during the day)

- Any bedwetting products (disposable liners, moisture detectors) your child is using and how effective they seem to be

- Any other symptoms your child seems to be experiencing

- Notes on any resources or information about bedwetting that you encounter that seems helpful

Health care professionals are busier than ever today and keeping such a diary can be a big help to a busy physician. Go over the notebook with your doctor and together look for patters, and possible causes. Get answers to the questions you have written down.

Keeping a diary can also be useful for you and for your child. If your child shows improvement (wetting every few days rather than once a night) you can show your child this improvement. If you yourself have any questions, you can easily refer to the resources and information you have collected in your notebook for more information.

Tip #42:   Explain any underlying problems

Sometimes, doctors will not pay attention to bedwetting once they have ruled out an underlying condition, because they assume that it is not a very threatening situation.

If your child's self-esteem, grades, or social development is affected by bedwetting, you need to let your doctor know because at that point bedwetting has moved from a non- threatening problem to a problem that is affecting your child's development. Discuss with your doctor the steps that must be taken to stop bedwetting or at least cope with the problems your child has developed as a result of it.

Tip #43:   Did your child's bedwetting develop at the same time as other symptoms?

If your child has developed bedwetting and snoring or extreme fatigue at the same time, you should mention this to your pediatrician.

In rare cases, something called Obstructive Sleep Apnea (OSA) may contribute to bedwetting. OSA means that some blockage - such as enlarged lymph glands called adenoids - block flow of air to the lungs.

In some cases, this problem causes snoring while for some children

OSA causes brief periods where breathing is entirely interrupted. OSA is thought to cause enough to seriously interfere with breathing. The most common cause of OSA is restless sleep, early morning headaches, and fatigue.

Some researchers have also linked this condition to bedwetting. Bedwetting caused by OSA is very rare, but can be treated, usually by removing the tonsils or adenoids. Your doctor can run a special test to determine whether your child's bedwetting is related to OSA.

Tip #44: Get a Second opinion

If you are not happy about your doctor's response regarding your child's bedwetting, don't be afraid to seek more help, possibly from a specialist. Get the care for your child that makes you feel comfortable. Every doctor has a different approach to child bedwetting. If your doctor is satisfied that your child will overcome the problem while you want some form of treatment, you may seek a physician who will help you.

Many parents are reluctant to seek a second opinion, even though they are not satisfied with a child's care. Many doctors are reluctant to recommend a child see an urologist or other professional because bedwetting is a problem.

However, you are the parent and you should take responsibility for your child's health. If your instinct tells you that something is wrong, seek a second opinion. Consider the following problems that can easily be mis-diagnosed or overlooked:

- bladder reflux - This illness can contribute to bedwetting and can require surgery to correct

- constipation - If your child does not empty his or her bowels regularly or completely, remaining waste can press down on the bladder and cause bedwetting.

- Malfunctioning of the urinary sphincter - The sphincter muscle is responsible for controlling urine flow. In those people who do not have a functioning sphincter, bedwetting is chronic and will not go away by itself.

- Kidney diseases - Some kidney diseases cause bedwetting as well as other symptoms. Without resolving the kidney problem, there is not much chance in successfully beating the bedwetting problem.

- Undiagnosed underlying problems - Some children may wet the bed due some serious problem such as abuse, diabetes, epilepsy, OSA, or other problems. If medical avenues are not carefully explored, these conditions will remain undetected and untreated, putting the child at risk.

Tip #45: Build a team.

There are many people in your child's life that can help ensure that bedwetting is a solvable and un-stressful problem:

- Teachers: You do not need to tell your teachers about your child's bedwetting, but you should be in contact with your child's instructors to make sure that your child's grades or social development is not suffering. An alert teacher can also often be your first alert of bullying or teasing that is taking place.

- Pediatrician: Your child's doctor should be one of your first stops when bedwetting becomes a problem, as your child's pediatrician can run tests to determine whether there are any physical or underlying causes behind the bedwetting.

- Therapists/Child Psychologists: If your child's grades, self-esteem, or social skills are affected by bedwetting, you may need to help your child develop a team of emotional support. Therapists and others can discuss your child's feelings with him or her and can help your child develop coping strategies for teasing and other problems.

- Pediatric nephrologist or urologist (kidney or urinary system specialist): In some children, a medical problem such as a badly working urinary sphincter can cause bedwetting. Kidney specialists and urologists can tell you whether your child's urinary system is fine or whether there is some underlying medical problem or physical problem behind the bedwetting.

If bedwetting persists very late (such as into adolescence) or is a nightly problem even by age eight or so, medical or physical reasons should be explored very carefully as they are a likely culprit.

Tip #46: Work with your team

You should choose the specialists who work with your child carefully, choosing those who seem to see the problem in the same light as you, and choosing those whose treatment options agree with you. When looking for health care professionals to treat your child's bedwetting, you will also want professionals who listen to you and your concerns.

Once you have found a team you trust, however, it is just as important that you work effectively with them. This means following instructions to the letter (asking for clarification when needed) and being very frank about other treatments you are using and about which treatments seem to be working and which do not.

Tip #47: Do Your Own Research

While a doctor can be very useful in helping you deal with your child's bedwetting, health care workers today are busier than ever and no one doctor can keep up with all the research and new information coming out each day. You may want to contact organizations such as the National Kidney Foundation or the American Academy of Pediatrics for more resources and then raise the information you find with your doctor.

You can contact some key resources about bedwetting yourself:

- The American Academy of Pediatrics (AAP) provides lots of useful information, and pamphlets about a variety of conditions, including bedwetting...

American Academy of Pediatrics (AAP)

141 Northwest Point Boulevard

Elk Grove Village, IL 60007_1098

Phone: (847) 434_4000

Fax: (847) 434_8000

Alternative address:

The American Academy of Pediatrics

Department of Federal Affairs

601 13th Street, NW

Suite 400 North

Washington, DC 20005 USA

Phone: (202) 347_8600

Fax: (202) 393_6137

Email: kidsdocs@aap.org

Web Address: http://www.aap.org

- The PottyMD is a great resource about toilet training and bedwetting. Since this groups focuses only on this problem, you are sure to get information that is pertinent to the topic. Many parents swear by this resource.

PottyMD

2216 White Avenue

Knoxville, TN 37916

Phone: 1_877_POTTYMD (768_8963)

Web Address: www.pottymd.com

- The National Kidney Foundation has recently launched a number of resources about bedwetting. Their website has lots of information and even video clips about the subject. Plus, if your child's bedwetting is caused by a kidney problem, this group can help you get information on that issue, as well.

National Kidney Foundation
30 East 33rd St., Suite 1100
New York, NY 10016
Phone: 1_800_622_9010

Web Address: www.kidney.org

- The National Kidney and Urologic Disease Information Clearinghouse provides all sorts of information about conditions that affect the kidneys and urinary system. Not surprisingly, they have several resources just about bedwetting.

National Kidney and Urologic Disease Information Clearinghouse
3 Information Way

Bethesda, MD 20892_3580

Phone: 1_800_891_5390

Web Address: www.kidney.niddk.nih.gov

- The Bedwetting Store carries a large selection of items relating to bedwetting. If you want to know about the latest items and devices that can help your child, consult this large online selection.

The Bedwetting Store

Phone: 1_800_214_9605

Web Address: www.bedwettingstore.com

- The American Academy of Child and Adolescent Psychiatry helps in distributing information about childhood psychiatry. It can be a useful resource if your child experiences undue upset because of bedwetting or if your child is experiencing secondary Enuresis caused by emotional trauma and needs treatment to overcome the problem.

American Academy of Child and Adolescent Psychiatry

Web Address: http://www.aacap.org

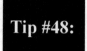

Tip #48: **Look for resources that can help you and your child understand what is going on.**

There are been a number of resources that are useful for parents:

- **Pamphlets**

  Doctor's offices, clinics, hospitals, and even pharmacies have pamphlets about various conditions - including bedwetting. These pamphlets can give you a general introduction to bedwetting, outline some commonly-used treatment options, and generally help you understand bedwetting.

  Since you will already have lots of information from this ebook, keep your eyes open for pamphlets about bedwetting that are designed for children. Written for children, these pamphlets tend to explain that problem in simple terms.

- **Videos**

  Pharmacies and some doctors or specialists have videos available that clearly discuss bedwetting. These videos use understandable language and plenty of visual information to inform parents and children alike about how the body works. It is sometimes useful to see pictures of the urinary system and to see the actual bedwetting treatments - seeing something visually can help with understanding.

- **Clinics or Specialists**

  Health care professionals can answer your specific questions about bedwetting and your child, and so should not be overlooked as possible sources of information. Medical professionals also often have access to all sorts of information and resources. Asking your medical professional "where can I get more information about this?" will generally give a treasure trove of reliable and accessible resources.

- **Articles**

The media writes about health issues all the time, and there is plenty of reason to pay attention. First, the media will often report on new treatments and products that may help your child. It may also help your child to see that a subject is written about and that others suffer from the same problem.

- **Online sites and groups**

Online resources are not always reliable, and so should be treated with some caution. Although some online resources about bedwetting are written by professionals, some are written about ordinary people who may know less about bedwetting than you do. Trust online information only from sources that you have confidence in.

On the other hand, online resources are very plentiful and are easy to look up. One type of online resource that many parents have found helpful is the online forum or chat. In this online area, parents can discuss health problems and health solutions.

Although, again, you have no way of knowing who you are speaking with and so need to exercise caution, many parents find that the sympathy and support they get from online groups helps them deal with a child who is wetting the bed.

Online speakers can also have some ideas about bedwetting and suggestions for specific problems (such as the best cleaners to use to eliminate odor or thrifty ways to save on sheets). As long as you use your common sense and some caution for online chat, you can find online forums informative and supportive.

- **Other parents or relatives**

Many families have at least a few people in the family who wet the bed. Talking to other parents about bedwetting often brings plenty of support and even some useful advice.

You should never discuss your child's bedwetting with another person without your child's knowledge. However, if your family is already aware of the problem you can often get useful information about what methods worked for children and what doctors or professionals in your area seem to have a high success rate in treating Enuresis.

Often, other parents and relatives will tell you information that others cannot know - the fact that a certain alarm is too high-pitched to work or that a certain brand of absorbent underpants has a special feature that make them useful. Those in the know often have great insights.

- **Pharmacists**

Pharmacists have plenty of information about all sorts of

ailments and treatments. If your child is taking any medications for bedwetting at all (including herbal or all-natural medicine) then you need to talk to a pharmacist to see whether the medication will interfere with any other medication (including over the counter drugs). Your pharmacist can help keep your child safe while he or she learns to control bedwetting.

Tip #49:	**Be cautious when evaluating bedwetting resources**

There are many sources out there about bedwetting. Unfortunately, there is also plenty of myths and misinformation about the subject, too. Make sure that you consider the following about any bedwetting resource you look at:

1) **Who wrote it?**

Was the author someone who knows about bedwetting?

2) **Why was it written?**

If something is written to convince you to buy something (an ad) you need to consider the claims more critically than if you were reading an article meant to inform rather than influence.

3) **Can the facts be verified?**

You should be able to look up the facts in the resource and find that other reputable bedwetting resources offer the same facts.

4) What is the publication date?

Older material may no longer be valid. New information is emerging all the time, so if you are using an old source, you are looking at information that may no longer be true.

5) Is there anything suspicious about this information?

If someone has basic facts wrong or seem to be offering a miracle cure that cures twenty illnesses, proceed with caution. Double-check the information the resource contains, at the very least.

Tip #50: Know what to expect.

Knowing what to expect when you take your child to the doctor with a bedwetting problem can make the trip less stressful for both you and your child. The first thing that the doctor will likely ask is about the bedwetting itself.

You may also be asked whether the child can control the bladder during the day (an answer of "no" means that the problem is not bedwetting per se but a problem controlling the bladder). Parents will also be asked whether the child has experienced any stress or changes lately and what the bedwetting is like (whether it is constant, when the child wakes up, etc.).

Finally, parent history and medical history will be taken, as some medical problems cause bedwetting, as do genetics (children with two parents who were bed wetters as children have a more than 76% chance of having a problem with wetting the bed themselves). Your doctor will likely check to see whether any medication or medical treatment your child is getting may contribute to the problem.

Once your doctor has evaluated the problem through questions and answers, he or she may decide that your child's age and medical history indicate no cause for concern and that waiting is the best solution. He or she may also order further testing.

One very common test is to determine whether the body can hold 200cc's of fluid. To determine this, the child is asked to hold urine for as long as possible and then have whatever urine is produced measured (often this is done by having the child urinate into a container so that the urine can be measured).

If the child cannot produce 200cc's then that is an indication that the bladder simply may not have developed enough. Doctors may also order urine or blood tests to see whether any underlying cause may be the problem.

6

BEDWETTING DEVICES AND TOOLS

Many manufacturers have created products to make bedwetting less traumatic. These devices and tools can make bedwetting less embarrassing and can make cleanup or activities such as camping easier. However, they should be used with treatment rather than a substitute for it as most of these products will not cure bedwetting themselves:

Tip #51:	Choose the right Moisture Detector Alarms

Moisture detector alarms are among the most effective tools in helping children overcome bedwetting. Unlike many of the devices and tools intended for children with Enuresis, alarms can actually treat bedwetting rather than just making the symptoms more bearable.

Moisture detectors are worn with underpants and the sensor of the alarm emits a loud sound when moisture is detected. The child can wake up and hurry to the bathroom in time. With use, the idea is to get the child to anticipate the alarm and wake up before any moisture is detected by the alarm. Within two or three months of nightly use, many children find that they can prevent all nighttime accidents and that they are actually getting up when their bladder is full and going to the bathroom.

Because moisture detection alarms are so effective in helping children overcome bedwetting, many manufacturers make them. However, all the different moisture detector alarms are not made the same.

If you choose the wrong model - one that makes your child uncomfortable or one that does not work well - the chances of success with the alarm are slim. You need a reliable and well-built alarm in order to help your child.

Signs of a good alarm include:

- **Reasonable price** - the alarm must be affordable

- **Comfortable to wear** - your child will need to wear this alarm nightly for a few months, anything that digs into your child, prevents sleep or has sharp edges could be detrimental. Plus, if your child hates wearing the alarm, he or she may not wear it often enough for the alarm to actually work

- **Right levels of sensitivity** - it is important that the alarm responds to small amounts of urine, so that the child can wake up in time to go to the bathroom. At the same time, an alarm that is too sensitive may be set off by night sweats, which will not only interrupt sleep unduly but will also make the alarm less successful in curing bedwetting.

- **Ease of use** - the alarm must be easy enough for your child to set and reset even in the middle of the night. Some alarms have a remote system that allows parents to reset the alarm from another room. This is useful for younger children.

- **Durability** - your child may drop the alarm in the night or may knock the alarm against the walls or bed during a restless night

- **Reliability** - The alarm must work each time urine is present, or it will be difficult to teach your child to solve bedwetting.

- **Hygienic design** - since the alarm will be in contact with urine, it is essential for good health that the alarm can be easily cleaned or disinfected after each use without its functioning being affected

- **Loudness** - The alarm should wake your child (and you, if your child tends to sleep through alarms). Some alarms come with adjustable sound levels, which can be very useful. Plus, some alarms allow children to be woken with vibrations rather than sound.

If you have large family, young children, or if your child shares a room, this can be a very useful feature. Plus, children not woken by sound may well be woken by movement, so this feature is very useful if your child has trouble being woken by an alarm.

- **Secureness** - Some alarms come with wireless technology to prevent tangling or pulled wires. This is a nice feature, but even a lower-end alarm is fine as long as it fits snugly with clips or some other secure fastener so that it will not dislodge even with nightly tossing and turning.

- **Size** - The alarm should be small enough to be worn with comfort, and should be the right size for your child. It should fit snugly enough so that it is not dislodged during a restless night

- **Simple power sources** - Most of these alarms work on batteries. Make sure any alarm you are considering buying uses batteries that are easily available. Stock up on batteries, as well.

- **Guarantee** - The manufacturer should be confident enough in the product to offer a full warranty or guarantee on the product. Remember: if the alarm does not work well each time, it will not be able to teach your child to overcome bedwetting. An alarm that is not consistent is useless.

- **Quality made** - The device should be sturdy and made with a design that shows some thought to patient comfort. The device should also be made to last.

Of course, you may not be able to try the device out in the store. However, the package label may at least give clues as to which of the above qualities are present in a product. Doctor or clinic reviews and recommendations from other parents can also help guide you to the alarms that have most of the above features.

Use Moisture Detector alarms effectively for success

Once you have chosen the best moisture detector alarm for your child, you will want to use it properly so that your child will actually learn to use the alarm to stop bedwetting.

The idea is not to use the alarm in order to alert that an "accident" has taken place. The idea is to get the child up quickly so that they will go to the bathroom in time - after some time with the alarm, many children are able to wake themselves up when they need to use the bathroom, without the use of the alarm. The idea is to get your child to anticipate the alarm and wake up before the alarm has gone off, when the bladder feels full.

Be sure to explain to your child the purpose of the alarm. Stress the idea of using the alarm to get up and go to the bathroom quickly when the alarm is heard. Better yet, practice with your child. Have the child activate the alarm with a damp cloth and then have the child hurry to the bathroom from his or her room.

Have your child practice setting the alarm and then resetting the alarm once he or she has gone to the bathroom. Practice with your child so that your child knows exactly what to do when the alarm goes off.

Make it easy for your child to respond to the alarm quickly. A hall light or other light source can help ensure that your child can move to the bathroom quickly and without injury when the alarm goes off at night. Make sure that the child can easily access a bathroom close to his or her bathroom.

If your child is a heavy sleeper, he or she may need help waking up when the buzzer goes off. If you hear the alarm, wake your child and help him or her to the bathroom. If your child has trouble waking up to the alarm, make sure that there is no noise in your child's room.

If your child sleeps in a noisy room, he or she may simply have become more adept at blocking out any noise, making him or her less likely to be woken up by noises of any type. Also ensure that your child goes to bed a little earlier than usual. Extreme tiredness caused by staying up too late will make it difficult for anyone to wake up for any alarm.

When using a moisture detection alarm, it is important to use the device faithfully each night until bedwetting episodes have stopped for at least a month. This may take a few months to accomplish, so patience is a desired trait when using this method to treat bedwetting.

Make sure that any bedclothes the child wears allow for proper use of the alarm. Thin underwear that allows a good grip for the clips that often come with the alarms, as well as a t-shirt to prevent tugging at wires, is often a good idea.

Even once your child has been dry using the alarm device, make sure that the problem has been resolved well. Some doctors recommend that the child drink more fluids before bedtime and continue wearing the device to ensure that the child really can wake up and go to the bathroom without "accidents." Even after the child is doing well, occasionally resorting to the alarm again can help "solidify" the learning, according to some experts.

Tip #53: Disposable urine absorbers.

Infants wear diapers to control the mess of urine flow. Now, there are disposable products designed for older children and even adults. These can help ensure a dry night and less mess to clean up. Today's products are made to be thin and discreet so that your child does not have to feel as though they are wearing diapers. These products are available through pharmacies and through medical supply stores.

However, even if your child wears these at night, be sure to pursue other options for actually treating the bedwetting. Disposable products are just a tool to make bedwetting less messy - they will not fix the problem.

These disposable systems are generally made to look like underpants, but they have liners of absorbent matter as well as top layers of plastic material to keep moisture away from the skin. For children who urinate only a little in their sleep, there are also liners that can be used with underwear.

Also be sure to keep your child's hygiene in mind while using these products. These products do keep moisture away from the skin but they can also be heavy and very warm when worn all night (especially in the summer). Teach your child to care for his or her skin to prevent sore skin.

Tip #54:　Reusable urine absorbers

There are urine stoppers that can catch urine during the night but which can be used again and again. These are less expensive than disposable products and can look either like underpants or like a combination of liner and underpants. Some parents prefer reusable urine absorbers because they keep sheets dry while still allowing a child to feel the wetness, which in some cases can wake the child up in time to go to the bathroom.

Used in this way, reusable urine absorbers such as underpants or liners can be used as part of behavior modification to cure bedwetting.

Tip #55:　Choose the right type of urine absorber.

Urine absorbers come in two basic types:

1) **Liners** - These are strips of absorbent material, covered with a stay-dry layer and underpinned with a waterproof layer. They are attached to the underpants with adhesive strips, slips, or bands of some sort. They can leak if a child urinates a larger amount, but they are often enough for children who wet only a little. These liners are quite discreet and can cause less skin irritation and discomfort. On the other hand, they can also dislodge during a restless night, not offering protection.

2) **Absorbent underpants** - There are underpants made of absorbent material that is covered in soft fabric that keeps the skin dry. The outside of the underwear is made waterproof and

may be covered in designs to make the underpants look more like regular "underwear."

These absorbent underpants can be very expensive, but come in many styles and sizes. The newer styles are thinner than ever and also more discreet (they do not create any tell- tale sound of crinkling). For small children, these underpants provide a large area so that leaks are less likely. These absorbers can also usually absorb more urine. These underpants can cause skin irritation as the skin cannot breathe very well. For this reason, it is important to choose the correct size.

You should choose an absorber that works for your child's situation and one that your child will not mind using. In some cases, it takes some trial and error for your child and you to find the absorber that is most effective and comfortable.

Tip #56: Mattress liners and mattress protectors

These products are placed under the sheets and keep the mattress free from moisture and stains. This can help protect a costly mattress and can make cleanup less of a hassle.

These are a good idea while your child wets the bed, as otherwise the smell of urine can linger in the mattress and make your child uncomfortable.

Also, without liners, each time your child wets the bed you will have to air out and dry the mattress, which can take all day. Liners make life easier for everyone in your family. Families who do not want to invest in expensive mattress liners and protectors can easily cover the child's bed securely with plastic wrapping (garbage bags, ponchos, any plastic material).

These have the advantage of being disposable as well as affordable, making clean up even easier. However, with these home-made innovations, you have to cover the mattress firmly as leaks may happen more readily with this solution, especially if you child is a restless sleeper. Store bought mattress liners are made to fit seamlessly and snugly over a bed, so that less leaking is possible.

Whatever sort of bed protection you use, make sure that all affected areas are covered. That means that if your child tosses and turns a lot, you should provide full mattress coverage as well as possibly pillow liners or protectors as well. Be sure to clean all protectors regularly (if they are not the disposable kind) to prevent odor.

Tip #57: Sleeping bag liners

These are more difficult to get than mattress liners, but they can make all the difference on camping trips and overnight stays at a friend's house. Check at on-line retailers, sporting goods stores, and medical supply stores. These liners keep the inside of a sleeping bag dry and odor-free thanks to an absorbent inner layer, a soft top layer and a waterproof lower layer that keeps the sleeping bad completely dry.

Tip #58: Those with chronic Enuresis often turn to catheters.

Catheters are medical equipment used to draw waste away from a body when a patient is very ill or unconscious. They are used by some patients with Enuresis. Traditional catheters will generally present a risk of infection and should not be used nightly.

Something called the "Texas catheter" fits over the genitals, is less invasive, and so is safer.

The idea is that the catheter gathers the urine into a disposable container, ensuring that the patient wakes up dry. Urine can be disposed easily, ensuring no clean up. Also, unlike absorbency undergarments, catheters draw the urine away more completely, reducing the chances of skin irritation or skin infection.

This is a bit of an extreme method, as it is not very comfortable and is certainly not discreet. However, it is used by some Enuresis patients who wet the bed each night due to a medical condition. If catheters seem like a solution to you, speak with a doctor or health care professional. Catheters are available through medical supply outlets, but if you decide to get one you may need to be trained to clean and use it properly and safely.

7

BEDWETTING ADVICE THAT HAS WORKED FOR OTHER PARENTS

Those who know a lot about bedwetting options, remedies and treatments are often those parents who have struggled with the problem with their own children. There are many alternatives or less-used bedwetting remedies used by parents to help treat the problem.

Some are backed by research; others are used simply because they work for some parents. At the very least, these tips are worth considering when you are trying to cope with bedwetting at your home:

Hypnotherapy

Hypnotherapy is an alternative treatment that uses hypnosis to treat bedwetting (Hypnotherapy is also used to treat a host of other ailments). The premise behind hypnotherapy is much the same as the idea behind behavior modification or visualization - the mind is used to control what the body does.

During hypnotherapy, a child will be hypnotized and then suggestions will be made (by the hypnotherapist's voice) that the child is able to control their bladder at night and can wake up in time to go to the bathroom. Hypnotherapy is safe and is generally used for older children, although there are hypnotherapists who work with younger children, as well. Some results can be seen in a few weeks.

If you decide to use hypnotherapy as a route, you need to investigate practitioners carefully, as in most states alternative healers such as hypnotherapists are not required to be licensed or otherwise controlled.

Get recommendations for a good hypnotherapist who has had success treating other patients of Enuresis specifically. Most health insurance does not cover this form of treatment, so get the best hypnotherapist you can so that your money is well spent on an effective remedy.

Tip #60: **Check Your Child's school bathroom and school drinking habits**

It sounds strange, but it's true - your child's habits at school may be contributing to problems at home. Some doctors have suggested that children do not drink very much during schooldays.

Partly, this is because children are given only short breaks and because beverages are not allowed in class. Children who do not drink enough in school may be dehydrated by the time they come home, meaning that they drink most of their daily fluids in the hours leading up to evening.

Plus, many children are shy about using bathrooms in public places, such as their school. This means that they may be waiting to drink and use the bathroom until they come home. This forces the body to take most of its water but also perform most of its voiding within a few hours, encouraging accidents in the night.

If your child has wet nights more often during the school week, school-related stress or poor drinking and bathroom habits may be the culprit. Ensuring that your child can drink and visit bathrooms regularly throughout the day can help ensure drier nights. Encourage your child to visit the bathroom at school and drink during school time. Discuss any concerns your child has about using the bathroom at school or drinking water at school. Try to remedy these problems.

Tip #61: Develop a bedtime routine.

Some parents have found that a steady bedtime routine helps some children relax and settle into sleep. A good night's sleep can help with bedwetting since the child is not going to sleep so tired that they will not wake up (even when their bladder is full) or so keyed-up that an accident is more likely to happen.

Plus, some parents have found that a steady routine helps to quiet the child and have the child prepare for bed in a good frame of mind. Some parents believe that just as the routine is established for bedtime, so the child's mind can accept a routine for getting up and going to the bathroom. At the very least, this method costs no money and is perfectly safe to use alone or with other remedies.

Tip #62: A teaspoon of honey

Some parents find that a teaspoon of honey taken orally morning and night helps prevent bedwetting. There is some controversy about this treatment, as some doctors insist that it does not work while some happy parents claim that it does. Research indicates that the substances in honey may help with water retention and help calm fears. More research needs to be done about these properties and their possible impact on bedwetting.

However, at the very least a teaspoon of honey at night and in the morning is not harmful in any way and can easily be used with other treatments.

Tip #63: Subliminal Suggestion

Ask your child if he or she dreams that she is urinating on the nights when he or she wets the bed. If your child does, have your child practice imagining waking up in the dream. Practice with your child, and have your child say "I have to wake up and go to the bathroom now" in the dream sequence. If your child can do this in their dream, they will wake up and have time to go to the bathroom. This is called "subliminal suggestion" and many parents find that this works like magic.

Tip #64: Homeopathy and natural remedies

If you can find a qualified homoeopath or alternative doctor in your area, he or she may be worth a try, especially if he or she has had success in treating bedwetting problems in the past. There are a number of natural medicines out there for treating bedwetting. You can easily and inexpensively buy them at the health food store.

However, a good natural healer or holistic practitioner can be a better choice as he or she will be qualified to tell which medications and natural treatments are effective. Many parents and their children have found success by pursuing this method.

If you decide to purchase herbal or homeopathic remedies of any kind, it is important that you read the ingredients very carefully to make sure that your child is not allergic to any of the substances. It is also a good idea to talk to your pharmacist to see whether any ingredients in the medication or treatment could interact with any substances your child is taking.

Remember: even remedies that are all-natural may contain ingredients that can be harmful or can cause allergic reactions in your child. Many parents have found help through natural or alternative tablets, pills, and other treatments, but you need to be cautious about what you give your child to ingest.

Tip #65: Chiropractors

Some parents have found help through chiropractic therapy. If you decide to opt for this route, make sure that you choose a qualified and recommended practitioner. It is best if you can find someone who has had experience in helping patients with Enuresis specifically.

Chiropractors work by manipulating the joints and the spinal cord in particular. It is thought that this manipulation helps to ease many conditions, including bedwetting. In fact, one recent study seems to prove that chiropractic treatment is beneficial for bedwetting prevention and treatment.

According to a study published in Journal of Manipulative and Physiological Therapeutics suggests that in some cases chiropractic treatment can help reduce bed wettings by half. In fact, the study found that chiropractic care helped more than 25% of subjects in the study make such dramatic improvement in their bladder control.

Chiropractic treatment is used by many people and when performed by a qualified practitioner is quite safe. It is even safe for children. However, you will want to find a practitioner with very good recommendations, as not all areas enforce strict controls on chiropractic practitioners.

8

PRE-TEENS, TEENAGERS, AND BEDWETTING

A small number of pre-teens and teens still wet the bed, and for these children, the problem can be quite upsetting. Since far few children in this age group wet the bed, Enuresis can be especially isolating for this age group.

Also, children at this age worry especially often about image and external appearance - what others think of them matters more, which can make a problem like bedwetting seem like a much greater concern. Pre-teens and teenagers are also more likely to be taking part in activities - such as dating and overnight trips - which are more affected by Enuresis. There are a few tips that apply specifically to pre-teens and teens who wet the bed:

Tip #66: Seek medical help aggressively.

By this stage, you should look for medical treatment aggressively, as it is clear that the old adage of "wait until he or she grows out of it" may not work in this case. Have a doctor do a full physical, and seek help from a urologist to find any medical conditions. If all seems well, then ask for tests to be run for rarer diseases. Then, seek a second opinion.

Tip #67: Keep an eye out for symptoms of trouble.

Teenagers and pre-teens may simply have a harder time dealing with bedwetting. The body or self-image of children in this age group is still developing, and something like bedwetting can affect self-esteem and self-image considerably.

At the same time, children in this age group tend to have more mobility and tend to be away from parental controls. Parents may not notice signs of problems until too late.

Parents will want to keep an eye out for:

- Signs of "acting out" - Older children may have access to drugs, alcohol, and other self- destructive habits (sex, stealing, cheating) that can become dangerous very quickly. Don't let a small problem become a big one.

- Signs of a poor body image - older children who feel as though their bodies are acting against them may feel uncomfortable in their bodies. This can lead to serious conditions such as anorexia and bulimia. Do not let your older child's bedwetting become a serious body problem

- Signs of depression or emotional upset - Signs such as loss of appetite, loss of interest in regular activities, and severe problems with sleep, school, and peers often indicates an emotional upset that needs to be handled.

- Drops in school marks - At the teen and pre-teen levels, school is very important as grades begin to count towards university acceptance and other life-altering events such as that. Any drops in grades could affect your child's future.

Tip #68: Treat any signs of trouble

The problem is that many teenagers and pre-teens are working very hard to become independent of their parents. Not only does bedwetting threaten this - which may make an older child withdraw more - but this independence may make it harder for parents to help a child, even when a parent notices the above signs of danger. If your notice the above signs, take your older child to doctor or therapist for help.

Tip #69: Use the fact that your children are older when treating bedwetting.

While treating pre-teens and teenagers with Enuresis is challenging in many ways, it also has its many advantages. Older children can take more responsibility for themselves and take care of the accidents they create with such precision that a parent might not even know that a problem still exists. Plus, older children can participate more fully in treatment as well - an older child can actually read this book and put some of the tips into work themselves!

9

SOME FINAL TIPS

As you finish reading this ebook, consider a few final tips that can help ensure drier mornings:

Tip #70: Be patient.

This is the advice most often given to parents about children's bedwetting. Although it is difficult advice to follow, it is also sound advice to a point. Since bedwetting often corrects itself in part or in full with time, a combination of some treatments and some patience is often necessary for success.

When trying new bedwetting treatments, it is often a good idea to give the treatments time to work, as well. There are no "instant" resolutions for bedwetting, and trying many remedies in rapid succession is not likely to work. In fact, it will not solve the problem but will often frustrate you as well.

Tip #71: Magnetic Therapy

New research has suggested than an alternative treatment called magnetic therapy has been shown useful in treating bedwetting in some children. A Korean University has found that children who were given treatment four times a week were less likely to suffer from Enuresis.

In this therapy, the child's pelvic floor is exposed to the magnetic therapy by having the child use a special magnetic chair. More research needs to be done on this, but it is thought that in the future, this therapy will be used to treat some children.

Tip #72: Check for rashes.

Once of the only physical effects of bedwetting is possible skin irritation and skin rashes cause by having urine so close to the body. This problem is most common in children who wear absorbent underpants or who wet the bed very frequently. In most cases, these rashes can be prevented with frequent mild washing and maybe with a soothing cream.

Tip #73: Check for Infection

Some children, especially younger children, though, may scratch at irritated skin. Left untreated, this can cause an infection, which causes even more unnecessary misery. If your child has an infection, you need to prevent scratching by keeping the child's nails clipped short.

You also need to visit your doctor for a medicated cream to treat the infection.

Since bedwetting can affect the skin, it is important to care for your child

's skin or teach your child to care for his or her skin carefully. Any signs of skin soreness should be treated promptly to prevent unnecessary suffering or infection. Infection is usually characterized by a wet, sore-looking skin area. Sometimes, yeast becomes active on the skin because of the moisture. When this happens, the skin may look bright red and spotted with pale flecks. For this infection, the doctor will often prescribe an anti- yeast medicated cream.

Tip #74: Consider Dry Bed Training

Some clinics offer a sort of intensive and advanced behavioral modification approach to bedwetting called "dry bed training." This can only be done by a professional, or with professional help, as it is quite complicated.

Children using this approach learn to stop wetting the bed through a combination of urine retention training, urine alarm system, self-correction, rapid waking training, positive affirmations and reinforcement, larger water intake, and toilet training. Some clinics and hospitals offer this program.

Your pediatrician or urologist may be able to help you find the training program nearest you. Because of the sometimes-high cost of this method, it is often restricted to those patients who have tried many other methods with no success.

Tip #75: **Take care of the problems the problem causes**

Even if no method is immediately available in treating bedwetting, or if no method seems to work, parents can help children cope with bedwetting more effectively, knowing that the problem will in most cases go away by itself. Even while you are waiting for methods to take effect, though, you may want to consider treating the problems that bedwetting causes.

After all, bedwetting itself is not dangerous or a huge problem. When children are upset by bedwetting, what they are often really reacting to are some of the problems associated with the problem. As a parent, you can help your child deal with these problems. When you do, your child will worry less about the problem and will be better able to handle the problem as you try treatment or as you wait for it to pass. Some of the most common problems that children face with bedwetting are:

Tip #76: **When your child thinks, "I'm embarrassed."**

Children often feel embarrassed by urinating at night, especially since it makes them feel that they are doing something embarrassing, hidden, or upsetting. For many children, processes like urination and body parts associated with urination are embarrassing.

Bedwetting just highlights all the embarrassment that children feel

74

about the whole topic.

You can help your child by repeatedly explaining that there is nothing to be ashamed of. Speaking frankly of body parts and processes can help, as can explaining frankly how the body creates urine and what happens when people wake up in time or don't wake up in time to urinate. This will demystify the process for your child and make it seem less of an embarrassing thing.

Tip #77:	**When your child thinks, "Does this mean that I'm 'bad'?"**

Many children think that not controlling their bladder at night makes then "bad." This may come from a few places. Children may hear adults saying "bad" to children who have had an accident (they may even see this on television). Children may also pick up on their parents' frustration with having to clean the sheets and bed after an accident.

The extra work a parent has to do, along with the frustration, can make a child feel guilty or even that he or she is unloved.

Reassure your child that urination is a body process and that it simply takes longer for some children to control their bladder. Continue to praise your child when he or she makes it to the bathroom in time, and never scold or punish your child for accidents. Make clean-up as easy on you as possible so that your child will not see you frustrated or upset as a result of bedwetting.

Tip #78:	When your child thinks, "This will never get better."

For children, time passes differently. A problem they have had for weeks may well seem forever. If they are the last children in their class or group of friends to wet the bed, they may feel that their problem will last "forever." Children who feel this may get discouraged and upset by the problem.

Reassure your child that the problem is temporary. If possible, have other family members discuss their own bedwetting experiences (and how they overcame it) with your child. Collect stories in the press of celebrities who wet the bed as children but outgrew it (celebrities will sometimes mention this sort of thing - or their biographers will - in interviews). This will help convince your child that the problem is only temporary.

Tip #79:	When your child thinks, "I'm not normal."

Children of a certain age worry very much about "fitting in." Anything that interrupts this often causes undue upset. Whether it is not having the "right" shoes or being different because of a medical condition, children who do not feel that they belong experience lots of stress. If your child thinks that he or she is the last 6-year-old (or 8-year-old or 16-year-old) that still wets the bed, your child may conclude that there is something "wrong" with them.

Have your doctor talk to your child and assure him or her that bedwetting is normal. Better yet, follow the advice above - have people that your child sees as normal talk about their childhood bedwetting. Once your child realizes that he or she is not "strange" by wetting the bed, some of the anxiety will decrease.

Tip #80: When your child thinks, "It takes so much time and work."

Ok, this is the cry of most parents who are faced with a child who wets the bed, but your child may also face anxiety about the upheaval that a "wet" night causes, especially if there are other people around to witness the fuss. If your child spends lots of time trying to work with bedwetting remedies or spends extra time cleaning up, he or she may also resent the time and work bedwetting takes up.

You can make bedwetting less of a problem for you and your child by making clean-up easier. Have your child wear absorbent underpants while trying to control bedwetting, or at least protect the bed and pillows with protective mattress liners. Keep extra bed linens and cleaning products in your child's room so that clean-up takes only a minute. Do larger loads of laundry to save some time, if you can.

Tip #81: When your child thinks, "I'm ashamed."

Many children are shamed by bedwetting - usually by the remarks made by a parent or another child. In general, a child is made to feel ashamed because those around him or her seem to make bedwetting a big deal or a sign of failure.

You can prevent your child from being ashamed by sticking to a "no big deal" attitude yourself. Make sure that your home is a no-tease zone and do not let other adults belittle your child. If a well-meaning relative starts to say something to your child about wetting the bed, praise your child publicly for doing well.

Saying something as simple as "Oh, John is doing much better with that now. We're all very proud of him" right to an adult who is making your child feel ashamed will make your child feel better. Positive reinforcement of any kind, in fact, will help your child. One of the best antidotes to shame is showing your child that you love and are proud of them.

Tip #82:	When your child thinks, "This means I'm lazy."

It is one of the myths about bedwetting that it is caused by laziness. Your child may hear this myth from another child or from an adult. It can make your child feel as though he or she is not "good enough."

Explain to your child how urination works and why some children cannot control their bladder until they are older. Point out all the things that your child does (chores, help, activities, school play) that prove that he or she is not lazy. Discuss what a myth is and explain why some people believe them.

Try saying something like, "Before, doctors didn't know why some kids wet the bed and some didn't, and someone thought that maybe it was because some kids were lazy. Now, doctors know that it's not true. Kids wet the bed because their bodies still need to grow in some ways, but some people haven't heard of this, and so they still believe the old idea."

This should help convince your child that the myth is not true.

Tip #83: When your child thinks, "This means I'm stupid."

Sadly, many people try to look for explanations in illnesses or conditions, trying to find out the "cause" behind something or trying to find out what something supposedly "means" rather than focusing on care or treatment. Your child may also be under the impression that the lack of bladder control "means something." Your child may assume that there is something wrong with his or her mind, as other kids have "learned" to stay dry.

When your child hears that the body does not wake the mind up to go to the bathroom - a common way Enuresis is explained to children - the child may assume that there is something wrong with their mind that is causing the bedwetting.

Praising your child's intellectual ability (putting good grades on the fridge or rewarding well done assignments) can help convince your child that he or she is intelligent. You can also take care to explain that children who wet the bed do not have anything wrong with their minds at all - they are just waiting for some body parts to grow up. This can hep reassure them that they are bright, that they just need to wait a bit longer to control their bladder.

Children who wet the bed may be teased by other children about the urine odor which may linger about their clothes and rooms. Even if this is not the case, many children associate urine with something "gross" or "dirty" and may feel disgust with their own bodies. If skin irritation develops, children may feel even dirtier, seeing marks of their bedwetting on their skin.

You can help your child feel clean by keeping their room and clothes clean and odor-free. Frequent washing, airing out of rooms and clothes, and use of a deodorizing cleaning product will usually keep odor away. Room sprays can also help. Using absorbent undergarments or sheet liners can help control odor and wetness. Also, help your child care for his or her skin or body and ensure that they always have fresh sheets and clothes on hand to use after an "accident."

You will also want to speak frankly with your child about urine and body waste. Explaining where it comes from and what it is can help your child overcome some of his or her disgust. Be sure that you do not encourage any of these negative feelings by wrinkling your nose or expressing distaste when cleaning after your child. Any other person in charge of cleaning up after your child should be taught the same.

When your child thinks, "I'm angry."

This is often a case of "why did this have to happen to me?" Children may feel that it is unfair that they have a problem with wetting the bed when others seem to have no problems sleeping a dry night. Some children may also be angry that other tease them about it. Anger often takes many forms, for withdrawal, to outbursts to violent flare-ups of anger with other children.

Getting your child to cool down is a top priority. Always have your child calm down quietly by himself or herself after a display of temper or defiance. Then, give your child a chance to tell their side of the story.

Of course, as a parent, you know that there are no answers as to why some things happen to some children and not to others. Explain that it is unfair that not everyone develops at the same time. Explain to your child some of the reasons behind bedwetting and sympathize with their anger.

Then, talk about what should be done when they feel anger. Discuss why anger happens and what can be done about it. If your child feels anger at home, you can try to encourage him or her to sit quietly, breathe deeply, and wait for the feeling to go away.

If your child is angry about being teased, try getting your child to act out what it said to him or her and have your child act out what he or she might say the next time something happens that is similar. You should not give your child excuses for expressing anger or violence, but you need to help your child deal with the feelings in a non-destructive way.

Tip #86:	When your child thinks, "I'm being teased."

Many children are teased at school for bedwetting. While adults know that most children will be teased for something at some point, and pay the problem no mind, teasing can be devastating to a child. Cruel nicknames such as "baby diapers" or worse can stick to a child and bring on the feelings of shame, anger, embarrassment, and worthlessness mentioned above, and this can be quite serious.

Have grown-ups talk to your child about what they were teased as a child (all the better if they were teased about bedwetting, too) and have them tell your child how the problem eventually got better.

Also, you may want to suggest to your child some things he or she can say when he or she is being teased. The best way to do this (especially with younger children) is to play make-believe. Have your child pretend to be the teaser, and pretend to be the child.

Have your child tell you where you are and have your child tease "you." Make the remarks you think are appropriate, suggest many things that the child could say. Then, switch roles. This game has several advantages:

- It makes the child feel in control, rather than helpless (which is the feeling teasing often creates)

- It allows the child to laugh at teasing

- It gives the child some idea of what can be said or done to teasers

- It builds the child's confidence

- It gives you a chance to evaluate the level and type of teasing your child experiences

- It opens communication with your child. Since the child feels free to tell you what is happening through "play acting" he or she may be willing to tell you what is happening in more detail, which can help you in deciding what to do about the teasing.

Tip #87: When your child thinks, "I'm being bullied."

One thing that you need to watch out for in terms of teasing is bullying. Bullying is teasing that has taken a more aggressive turn. In many cases, it escalates with time and can include actual physical violence. Some children have even died at the hands of bullies who have targeted them.

Sometimes, it can be hard to tell when teasing has taken the turn to bullying, but in general if your child seems traumatized by the teasing he or she is getting at school, you should treat the teasing as bullying.

Also, if there is any physical aggression or any threats then the situation is certainly bullying. Bullying is a crime in many locations and needs to be brought to the attention of parents, school authorities, and possibly authorities as well. Bullying needs to be taken seriously at once, as it can very quickly get completely out of hand.

Of course, adults know that bullying and teasing are not caused by bedwetting - child bullies will target any child who seems unsure of themselves and any child who displays signs of being "different." However, bedwetting can be a sign of difference and can affect a child's self-esteem to the point where they do make a target for other children.

In some cases, therapy or visits to a counselor can help your child get the social skills needed to deal with teasing. In other cases, more help is needed, especially if bullying is an issue.

In many cases, trying to deal with the bully's parents has little effect, as not all parents can control what their children do outside the house. Moving away is also not always effective, as teasing may simply continue at the new location.

Tip #88:	**When your child thinks, "I feel like a baby."**

For children, acting "grown up" is important, partly because children look up to adults so much and often want the power and control, they think that adults have. For a child who wets the bed, though, there is a sense of the opposite feelings - lack of control, and lack of power. Children who wet the bed may feel powerless.

Many children may worry that they are acting "babyish," especially since this is one of the first accusations leveled against bed wetters on the playground. For an adult, being called a "baby" may not be a big problem, but it can feel like a devastating problem to a child, especially a younger one who may see being a "baby" as being left behind while others in the same age group "grow up."

To offset these feelings, make sure that your child understands that children of all ages - even children who are older - wet the bed. It is truly not a problem of age, but a problem of bladder control, and it can affect people of all ages. While children do eventually "outgrow" the problem in many cases, many children your child would consider "grown up" still face the same problem.

Tip #89:	When your child thinks, "I hate having a big secret."

Most children try to keep bedwetting a big secret, as they are fearful that others will find out. However, having a large secret can affect the way your child's relationships and can leave him or her feeling lonely. Having a large secret is isolating, to say the least.

Plus, your child has all the stress of knowing that the secret may be exposed. The older a child is, typically the more effort will go into keeping bedwetting a secret. Among the things that children will do to keep bedwetting a secret are:

- Avoiding sleep overs, camping trips, and other events for fear of being "found out."

- Avoiding bringing home other children, out of fear that someone in the home will "tell."

- Adopting an "I don't care" attitude or acting aloof in order to

85

avoid getting close to others.

- Avoiding making friends.

- Staying up all night on camping trips or during sleep overs in order to prevent accidents.

- Teenagers may avoid dating.

- All children may avoid attention or notice by refusing to try to excel at school or activities.

- Acting in a "tough" or self-destructive way so that no one will guess the "truth."

Your child may put themselves through a lot to prevent others from finding out that they wet the bed. This can create a lot of tension in the home and also ensures that your child will not make close friends.

Worse, your child may give up fun trips or exciting events just out of fear of accidents. This is limiting. You certainly don't want your child to grow up fearfully or in great tension.

Generally, whether your child chooses to tell others about their bedwetting or not is up to them. You should never tell someone else about your child's bedwetting - the child should be able to decide who to trust and who not to trust.

Telling anyone - even a well-meaning teacher or relative - without the child's consent is a recipe for disaster, especially if your child is keeping the problem a secret. Your child may simply cease to trust you and will likely feel more fearful as well as resentful.

However, you can help your child open up to others by showing your own acceptance of the problem. If you treat the problem matter-of-factly and with sensitivity, your child may start to trust that others will, too.

Plus, you should encourage your child to spend time with others as much as possible. Discuss things such as camping trips or other events ahead of time and discuss with your child how he or she could handle bedwetting or the possibility of accidents in such a situation.

In a way, your child may be relieved when his or her secret is finally revealed. However, it can also be a very traumatic time, especially if the "truth" is met with teasing or disapproval.

You may want to speak to your child about what he or she would feel like if someone did find out. Discuss the responses that your child expects from others and then suggest more gentle responses that may be possible, too. Talk with your child about things that he or she could say to negative or insensitive comments.

Tip #90: When your child thinks, "I don't want to go anywhere."

Many children who wet the bed show less interest in spending lots of time with others, especially if they are teased or are trying to prevent others from learning about their bedwetting.

This can lead some children to isolate themselves and can also lead to such a low state of self-esteem and happiness that children will stop their regular fun activities as well - even if those activities do not involve sleeping over or even other people. This can be a serious sign of upset and should be taken seriously.

A lack of interest in what is happening can be a big problem of bedwetting. Children can become unenthusiastic, depressed, listless, and apathetic, leading to lack of activity and increasing depression.

You can try enticing your child's interest in new things by encouraging him or her to take part in new activities that seem appealing. Offer support for activities that your child has done in the past that he or she has excelled in, and offer some part of an activity as a treat. For example, if your child has always liked baseball, buy him or her a new glove or a baseball card to revive interest. If nothing seems to work and apathy lasts longer than a week or so, take your child to a doctor to make sure that no physical problem or serious emotional trauma are causing the disinterestedness.

Tip #91: When your child thinks, "I feel insecure."

No child will simply come right out and say it that way, but there are many signs that a child is feeling that way on some level. Children who feel this way will often try to be loud to garner more attention or will be quieter and try to attract as little attention as possible. Children may bully others or attract bullies as a target. They may cling to the home, fearful of venturing anywhere else. They may become quite clingy and demanding in all sorts of ways.

Insecurity is a bigger problem than many thinks. It can lead to experimentation with drugs in older children who want to "fit in" and it can lead to a host of destructive behaviors, even in younger children.

It can prevent children from trying new things and hold them back from excelling. It can also lead to image problems and feelings of unhappiness or even depression.

Building self-esteem in children is a long road, but it can be done. Start by praising your child for the things that he or she does right. Also encourage your child to take part in activities or try things outside the home. Often, when a child accomplishes something "all by themselves" the pride of the success will outweigh all the positive praise possible, as it creates a real feeling of accomplishment.

Tip #92: When your child thinks, "What will others think?"

Children often worry most about other people's reactions rather than about actual bedwetting. Put another way, if there was no one else around, bedwetting would be far less stressful for a child as there would be no one else to know about the problem. Many children imagine what others would say, and the imagination is always worse than the reality. Or, your child may have had one or two experiences of being teased for the problem and now is fearful that others will react in a like way.

Either way, worrying what others will think makes a much bigger problem out of bedwetting. Such anxiety also puts lots of stress on a child, often unnecessarily. You can help your child overcome this problem by discussing with your child possible reactions people might have to the bedwetting and discussing what could be said in response.

If someone accuses him or her of being a baby, for example, you child can point out that lots of older kids wet the bed or tell the teaser that bedwetting is not about being a baby, but rather a condition. Be sure to discuss possible nice or sensitive things people could say, too, so that your child is not just imagining the worst.

If your child is hesitant about other people's reaction because he or she has already had a negative experience, you will have to work a bit harder. Talk to your child about the incident, and consider why someone would have a bad reaction (Could they have been ignorant about bedwetting? Could they have been having a bad day and just taken it out in that way? Could they just be mean-spirited, saying something unpleasant about anyone, whether they wet the bed or not?).

With your child, discuss what the child would do or say in the same situation. Then, talk about any positive experiences the child has had with people learning about his or her bedwetting and discuss possibly kind things that people could say once they find out.

This sort of role playing is very effective in having your child feel in control of situations where people learn about the bedwetting. Often, the most frightening thing about someone's reaction to us is that we cannot control the reaction. Imagining what to say gives your child some of that control. Also, imagining or remembering positive reactions will take your child out of the mind frame that all reactions will be bad.

Tip #93: When your child thinks, "This makes home feel terrible."

Bedwetting affects not just the child afflicted with Enuresis, but rather the whole family. In some cases, children may resent the home or may feel that their problem creates an unpleasant atmosphere at home.

Parents may disagree over the treatment options; siblings may feel jealous of the attention the child receives or may tease their sibling over the problem. The child may also come to associate his or her bedroom with nighttime discomfort. There are many ways that bedwetting can affect the home, and few of them are pleasant.

The best way to counteract this problem is to work together as a team. Everyone in the family should be included in decisions that affect the whole household (decisions such as changing a sleeping room so that one child will be closer to the bathroom, for example).

You should also try to make home as un-tense as possible. Make bedwetting less of a family upheaval by making clean-ups easy and by making the child affected help with some clean-up. Also, make sure that you have everyone in the household agree to no teasing. Creating a serene home environment is helpful for everyone affected by bedwetting.

Tip #94: Take it one step at a time.

You can't expect your child to stop wetting the bed overnight. For many children, the process takes months or years, and even then, the occasional "accident" can happen. Take things one step at a time, slowly helping your child and celebrating successes (such as a week or a record three days dry in a row). Rushing will not accomplish anything and will just put unnecessary pressure on the child.

Tip #95: Stay organized.

Try one method at a time and carefully record on paper how effective it is (the easiest way to do this is to mark off which nights are dry and which are not so that you can see if there is an improvement). If you try several methods at once, you will have no way of knowing which remedies are working and which are not.

Tip #96: Give a method time to work before tossing it aside.

In general, most methods should give you at least some minor result within two weeks. However, some methods may take longer to show effect. Do not be in a rush to try every method. The goal is to help your child, and you do not want to overlook a method that would work just because you want "instant" answers. If you have not seen improvement in a few weeks, though, by all means try some other method to see whether your child can find relief some way.

Tip #97: Combine some tips for best results.

Where no interaction is a factor, try combining tips to get great results. For example, you can often combine natural or homeopathic alternative therapies with behavior modification. Most tips work well with comfort tips such as protecting sheets. Of course, you do not want to combine medications, but combining behavioral modification with some natural supplement or dietary changes may do the trick.

If you are going to be combining remedies, make sure above else that the two methods will not be dangerous together. Then, introduce each therapy to your child one at a time so that your child can get used to each treatment and so that you can observe any adverse effects.

Tip #98: Try simplest methods first.

You want the best for your child, but the best is not always the most complicated or high-tech method. With young children, especially, simplest methods are best. They also tend to be the most effective. For example, low-cost moisture detector alarms have very high rates of efficiency, even when compared to high-priced training. Look for inexpensive treatments that are simple enough for your child to understand. If those are ineffective, then you can move on to other methods.

If you start with the most complicated gadgets and solutions, you may find yourself spending a lot money than you planned if that first treatment does not work. Plus, if you put too much faith in the latest high-tech solution and your child's problem is not resolved, both you and your child will have to deal with the disappointment.

Keep your expectations realistic (gradual improvement over time) and keep your solutions simple. Both your child and your wallet will thank you for it.

Tip #99: Understand all risks before you begin

Some methods of bedwetting treatment have almost no risks (think of the honey cure or visualization, for example). Some are risky when administered improperly (alternative or holistic medicine, chiropractic therapy) and some are risky (all medications carry risks of side effects). Make sure that you understand what can go wrong with each treatment before you begin it. Make sure that you can cope with the eventuality if it happens.

Of course, you should try low-risk options (behavior modification, for example) before higher risk options (such as medication). It makes sense to keep your child safe, especially if the bedwetting issue can be resolved with no possible injury. Move onto riskier methods if the low-risk methods do not seem to be working after a few weeks.

Tip #100: Keep your eye on the big picture

As you browse through this ebook, you may be excited that so many possible solutions exist for bedwetting. However, do not focus on these tips so much that you lose track.

Your main goal is to make your child feel comfortable and to help your child feel happy.

If you can do this with methods for getting rid of bedwetting, then great. However, putting the focus on your child first means that you will not lose track of your child's comfort level as your try to help your child stop wetting the bed.

Tip #101: Love your child

If you are reading this book and trying to help your child, then you likely don't need to be told - but does your child? Children who are experiencing bedwetting and treatment for the problem often experience great upheavals of emotions. They need your love more than ever, and they especially need to be told that they are loved - right now. Being affectionate and loving with your child will help reassure your child more than anything that he or she is still loved and accepted. This can help give your child the strength to get over teasing and the other problems associated with bedwetting.

Don't just assume your child knows you love them - especially if you have been short- tempered with them concerning bed wetting or bedwetting treatment. Tell them.

10

CONCLUSION

Now that you have pondered more than one hundred ways to help your child with bedwetting, the time has come to choose which methods to use in helping your child.

You may have chosen some methods to put into practice already or you may be wondering where to begin. You will notice that the methods of dealing with bedwetting fall into a few broad categories:

- **Time and patience:** Often the most-recommended method, this means that parents and children wait until the body on its own learns to stop losing bladder control at night. This can be a frustrating method, but tends to be an effective one, as most children tend to outgrow the problem on their own with time. All methods require at least a small dose of time and patience to work.

- **Behavior Modification:** This method works by trying to "teach" the body to wake up in time in order to go to the bathroom. Various methods are used in this treatment. Moisture detector alarms, making bathroom access easier, visualization, and other techniques are all used.

- **Reduction of Mess or Problem:** Some parents simply see bed wetting as a natural part of childhood, and work to simply reduce the mess and inconvenience. A number of products on the market today exist to help with this goal, including mattress liners, sleeping bad liners, disposable absorbent underpants, non-disposable absorbent products, and many others.

These can all make mornings more pleasant until the child learns to sleep "dry." In many cases, you should use one of these methods no matter what method you are using, as "accidents" may occur.

- **Medical Treatment:** Some parents seek doctor help with bedwetting. This can be a good idea if a parent suspects an underlying cause may be the real problem behind bedwetting. Even if the cause is not medical, doctors can prescribe medication that can control bedwetting.

- **Holistic Treatment:** A number of alternative treatments exist which help children with bedwetting. Eating honey, hypnotherapy, and other such treatments have been found effective by some parents, even though these treatments do not work for everyone and even though in some cases not much research has been done about the efficacy of these treatments.

- **Proxy Treatment** - Rather than treating the problem, some parents choose to treat the problems caused by the problem. This can mean helping a child cope with teasing or clean-up or discomfort. The idea is that if the problem is more bearable, the child will be able to wait for the problem to clear up on its own.

Also, proxy treatment acknowledges that it is often not bedwetting itself that is a problem, but rather it is the problems caused by it that seem unbearable.

Most parents use at least a few treatments, if not several. They may use a few remedies to control the mess of bedwetting, for example, and use others to actually resolve the problem. Different parents use different methods, just as different doctors will suggest different ways for dealing with bedwetting. Whatever treatment system you choose for your child should have a few basic qualities. It should:

- Be accepted by the child

- Not make the problem worse

- Be safe

- Be effective

- Be affordable for your family

- Cause a minimum of disruption in the home

- Not require so much time that other family activities or responsibilities suffer

- Be a system that both the child and the parent feel comfortable with

- Suit your child's and family's specific circumstances

- Not interfere with normal child development and activities

There are many treatments and tips throughout this ebook that may have these qualities for your case. Choose those tips that make sense to you and give them a try to see if they help. Many parents have found help by following the advice on these pages, and now that you have the tips in this ebook, you will be able to effect similar success stories with your own family.

Mornings will seem much nicer when your child is well rested AND happy, so go back, choose the tips you want to try and start your way to calmer wake-ups.

CPSIA information can be obtained
at www.ICGtesting.com
Printed in the USA
LVHW080537180422
716440LV00014BB/1085

9 788367 314046